THE ART AND SCIENCE OF LONGEVITY

THE COMPREHENSIVE GUIDE TO HABITS THAT MAKES THE BODY NOT TO DIE.

Barrett S. Moulton

Copyright © 2023 Barrett S. Moulton

All rights reserved. No part of this book may be reproduced, stored, or transmitted in any form or by any means, without the prior written permission of the publisher, except in the case of brief quotations embodied in critical articles or reviews.

TABLE OF CONTENTS

INTRODUCTION
- Theories of Aging
- The importance of longevity and healthy aging.

CHAPTER 1: THE FOUNDATIONS OF LONGEVITY
- Understanding the aging process Genetics and Longevity.
- Role of lifestyle Factors in Longevity

CHAPTER 2: NUTRITION AND LONGEVITY
- The importance of healthy diet for longevity
- The best foods for Longevity
- Role of Supplements in Longevity

CHAPTER 3: EXERCISE AND LONGEVITY
- The Benefits of Exercise for Longevity
- Types of Exercise that promote Longevity
- Tips for staying Active

CHAPTER 4: SLEEP AND LONGEVITY
- The Importance of Sleep for Longevity
- How to Improve your Sleep Habits

CHAPTER 5: STRESS MANAGEMENT AND LONGEVITY
- The Effects of Stress on Health
- Stress Management Techniques

CHAPTER 6: SOCIAL CONNECTIONS AND LONGEVITY
- The Role of Social Connections in Longevity
- How to maintain connections as you age
- The Benefits of Volunteering and giving back for longevity

CHAPTER 7: ENVIRONMENTAL FACTORS AND LONGEVITY
    How Environmental Factors Can Impact longevity
    Tips For Reducing exposure to harmful toxins
    The Benefits of Living in a healthy Environment For Longevity

CHAPTER 8: LONGEVITY AND TECHNOLOGY
    The Latest advancements in Longevity research
    How technology is changing the field of longevity
    The future of Longevity and Healthy Aging

CHAPTER 9: CONCLUSION

21 DAYS HEALTHY HABITS JOURNAL

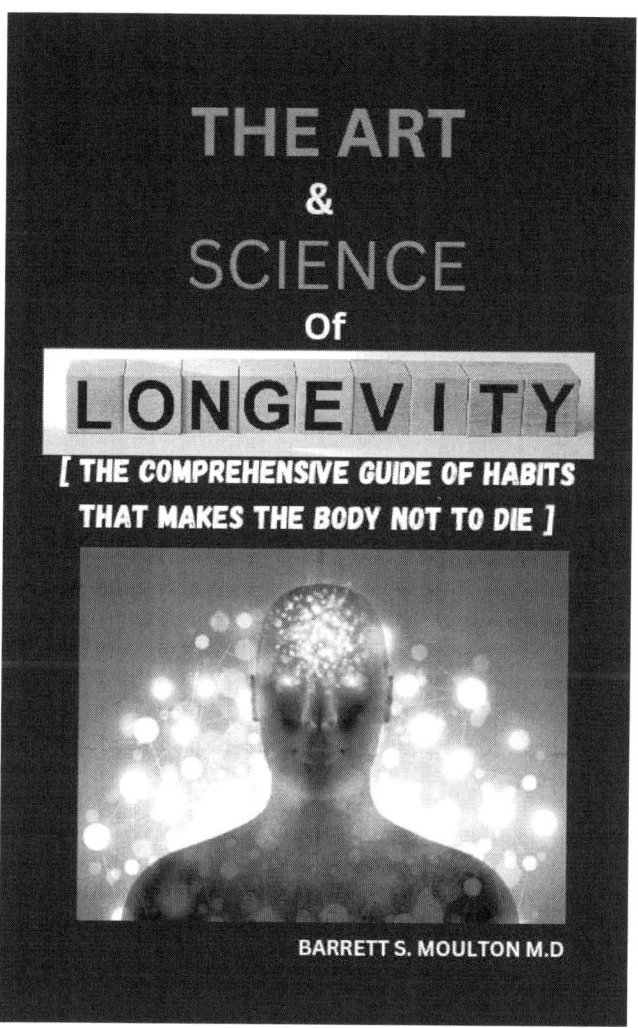

INTRODUCTION

In recent years, the value of longevity and healthy aging has become more and more clear. People are living longer than ever because of developments in medical research and a better grasp of how the aging process works. Additionally, as we strive to preserve our quality of life as we age, the emphasis on healthy aging has grown more significant. Longevity and healthy aging are important because they prolong our quality of life, lower our chance of developing age-related illnesses and disabilities, and allow us to continue working and participating in our communities.

The term "longevity" refers to how long someone lives, and the phrase "healthy aging" refers to the process of aging in a way that promotes both physical and mental health. In other words, it is the capacity to age devoid of the onset of infirmity, chronic sickness, or cognitive deterioration. According to research, a combination of physical activity, social interaction, a nutritious diet, and mental stimulation can help to promote healthy aging. In addition to lowering the risk of depression and loneliness, physical activity is crucial for preserving physical health, strength, and flexibility. Mental stimulation can assist to avoid memory loss and cognitive decline, and appropriate eating is vital for giving the body the nutrients it needs to be strong and healthy.

Theories of Aging

Aging is a universal, innate, and continuous process. Since the time of the ancient Greeks, theories of aging have been contested, and academics now believe that no single explanation can adequately explain all facets of aging. Instead, it is possible to combine numerous ideas to explain different facets of the complicated phenomenon known as aging.

What causes us to age? Recently developed biological ageing ideas have emerged from scientific research. What causes cellular aging. This movie examines 12 current theories about the causes of aging, including DNA genome damage, telomere shortening, epigenetic problems, protein misfolding, cell senescence, stem cell exhaustion, glycation, inflammation, MTOR pathways, and Sirtuins (longivity genes). Later on, several of these theories are described.

One way to think about aging is as a series of events that happen from conception to death. All types of ageing theories aim to examine and explain the various facets of aging.

Biologic: Interested in finding answers to fundamental concerns about the physiological processes that all living things go through over the course of their lives (Hayflick, 1996).

Sociological: examining the roles and connections that people make in later life.

Psychological: Affected by genetics and sociology; deals with how a person reacts to social situations that are appropriate for their age.

Moral/Spiritual: Examine how people attempt to justify their existence.

Ageing Biological Theories

The goal of biological theories is to provide explanations for the physiological changes that all living things go through as they get older. The goal of this research is to identify these triggering elements that initiate the actual aging process in organisms. These age-related alterations occur independently of any pathogenic or environmental impacts.

THEORIES PROGRAMMED

According to the theory of "Programmed Longevity," aging is the result of certain genes being turned on and off one at a time. Senescence is the point at which age-related deficiencies become apparent.

Endocrine Theory, which holds that biological clocks regulate the rate of aging by way of hormones.

According to the immunological theory, the immune system is designed to deteriorate with time, which makes people more susceptible to infectious diseases, aging, and death. check out immunosenescence

According to the theory of "Programmed Longevity," aging is the result of certain genes being turned on and off one at a time. Senescence is the point at which age-related deficiencies become apparent.
Endocrine Theory, which holds that biological clocks regulate the rate of aging by way of hormones.
According to the immunological theory, the immune system is designed to deteriorate with time, which makes people more susceptible to infectious diseases, aging, and death. See Theories of Immunosenescence Damage or Error.

FREE RADICALS THEORY:

According to the free radical theory, the primary cause of cellular aging is the steady buildup of oxidative cellular damage. This theory has changed over time to emphasize the importance of mtDNA mutations caused by free radicals and the buildup of mtDNA deletions. Given that the electron transport chain, a major source of free radicals, is close to the mtDNA, it is hypothesized that the mutations will encourage mitochondrial malfunction and, as a result, boost the generation of free radicals in a positive feedback loop. It is well known that diet, way of life, drugs (including alcohol and tobacco), radiation, etc., all speed up the body's generation of free radicals.
Error theory: founded on the notion that mistakes can happen during DNA synthesis or transcription. These mistakes keep happening, and eventually they cause systems to not perform as well as they should. These occurrences are responsible for the organism's aging and demise (Sonneborn, 1979).
The Glycosylation Theory of Aging is another name for the Cross-Linking Theory. According to this view, numerous issues are brought on by the binding of glucose (simple sugars) to protein, a process that takes place when oxygen is present. Once this binding has taken place, the protein is impaired and can no longer function as effectively. Living a longer life will increase the likelihood of oxygen interacting with glucose and protein, and known problems of cross-linking include senile cataract and the development of rough, leathery, and yellow skin.

The Theory of Neuroendocrine: This idea, which was initially put forth by Professor Vladimir Dilman and Dr. Ward Dean, elaborates on wear and tear by concentrating on the neuroendocrine system. The hypothalamus, a brain-based gland about the size of a walnut, controls the release of hormones through a complex network of biochemicals in this system. The hypothalamus regulates a number of chain reactions that tell other glands and organs when and how to release hormones, among other things. As a reference to the total hormonal activity, the hypothalamus also reacts to body hormone levels. However, as we age, the hypothalamus loses its ability to precisely regulate, and the receptors that take in certain hormones become less sensitive to them. As a result, many hormones become less secreted as we age and become less effective (when compared unit to unit) as a result of receptor downgrading.

The Ageing Membrane Theory: This idea holds that the cell's ability to transport chemicals, heat, and electrical processes becomes impaired as it ages. The cell membrane gets less lipid (less fluid and more solid) as we age. This makes it more difficult for it to carry out routine tasks, and in particular there is a poisonous buildup.

The Theory of Decline In every cell of every organ, there are organelles called mitochondria that produce energy. They do this in the many energy cycles that involve nutrients like Acetyl-L-Carnitine, CoQ10 (Idebenone), NADH, certain B vitamins, and others. Their main task is to produce adenosine triphosphate (ATP).To stop and slow down aging, the mitochondria must be strengthened and protected. The aforementioned nutrients, as well as ATP supplements themselves, can enhance.

EMERGING THEORIES:

The neuroendocrine system regulates a number of critical processes that are essential to growth and development. This is known as the pacemaker theory. The hormones DHEA (dehydroepiandrosterone), melatonin, and the hypothalamus are being studied for their roles in the aging process. Over the course of a person's lifespan, DHEA production by the adrenal glands declines. Laboratory mice that get this hormone live longer, have stronger immune systems, and look younger. These mice also consumed less food, indicating that the effect of calorie restriction may be seen in DHEA-fed mice. A hormone called melatonin is produced by the pineal gland and functions as an immunological booster, a potent antioxidant, and a regulator of biological cycles. From just after puberty until old age, the body produces much less melatonin.

Caloric Restriction and the Metabolic Theory of Aging: This theory contends that all creatures have a finite metabolic lifetime and that those with a greater metabolic rate have shorter life spans. This is supported by research demonstrating that some fish have higher life spans in colder water than in warm water. Numerous studies on the effects of calorie restriction on rodents have shown that it lengthens life and postpones the onset of age-dependent illnesses.

DNA-Related Studies: Regarding DNA and the aging process, two breakthroughs are now taking place: One, as they continue to sequence the human genome, scientists are uncovering specific genes that contribute to aging Two, the identification of telomeres, which are found at the ends of chromosomes and may serve as biological clocks for cells (Hayflick, 1996)

SPIRITUAL THEORY:
Look at the person's attempts to justify and explain their existence. Research on the relationship between spirituality or religion and health is debatable. Some people think it is unscientific to examine religion along with other health factors. Despite this, it appears that spiritual affectations become more pronounced as people age, and the scientific community needs to investigate the relationship between religion, spirituality, and health in order to completely understand how spirituality affects aging.

Theories of ReligionSpiritual.jpg
Look at the person's attempts to justify and explain their existence. Research on the relationship between spirituality or religion and health is debatable. Some people think it is unscientific to examine religion along with other health factors. Despite this, it appears that spiritual affectations become more pronounced as people age, and in order for the scientific community to completely grasp spirituality's impact on aging, the relationship between religion, spirituality, and health needs to be explored.

Biologically and sociologically influenced psychological theories focus on how a person responds to the demands of his or her age[3]. Psychological theories predate all other known theories of aging. They consist of:

According to the Human Needs Theory, human conduct is driven by needs as people get older. Specifically, physical, security and safety, love and belonging, self-worth, and actualization.Life-Course (Lifespan Development) Theory: Developed in the 1980s by behavioral psychologists who decided to use the idea of "life course" rather than personality development as the foundation for aging research. According to this view, the stages of life may be predicted and are produced by objectives, relationships, and personal values. The connection of the individual and society is the main theme of this ideology.

According to the disengagement theory, many of a person's connections to other people in society end and those that remain change in quality with time. Withdrawal might be partial or complete and can be started by society or the elderly person. Elderly folks have been seen to be less engaged in life than younger adults. People grow more removed from society as they get older, and they form new kinds of connections with it. There is evidence that older individuals in America are forced to retreat by society, whether or not they like to. Some claim that this hypothesis fails to take into account the significant proportion of elderly people who remain active in society. This idea is acknowledged as the first official theory that made an effort to explain the aging process.Activity Theory: explains how people mature psychosocially. highlights the value of constant social interaction. suggests that a person's self-concept is tied to the roles that they play; for example, retiring may not be as bad if the individual actively maintains other responsibilities, like familial, recreational, volunteer, and community duties. A person must fill in for duties that are lost as they get older in order to keep a positive sense of self. The type of activity does crucial,according to research just as it does for the people.

The importance of longevity and healthy aging

Longevity and healthy aging are ideas that have been around for many millennia and are frequently regarded as indicators of excellent health and welfare. Understanding the value of longevity and healthy aging is becoming more and more crucial as life expectancy rises and the global population expands.

Simply said, longevity is a measurement of a person's life expectancy. It is the anticipated lifespan of an individual. Maintaining one's physical, mental, and social well-being as one ages is known as healthy aging. Physical and mental exercises work together to keep a person's cognitive and physical abilities sharp as they age.

Longevity and proper aging have several advantages. The biggest advantage is a better quality of life. People frequently become less active and lose muscular mass as they get older. Overall quality of life, including physical and mental health, may suffer as a result. However, people cankeep their muscle mass and general health as they age by staying active and eating a good diet.

The danger of contracting diseases and chronic conditions is decreased, which is another important advantage of longevity and healthy aging. The likelihood of contracting illnesses including cancer, heart disease, and diabetes rises as people get older.

CHAPTER 1: THE FOUNDATIONS OF LONGEVITY

Understanding the aging process Genetics and Longevity.

Genetics, environment, and lifestyle all have an impact on how long people live. With major increases in the availability of food and clean water, better housing and living circumstances, decreased exposure to infectious diseases, and more access to medical treatment, environmental changes starting in the 1900s dramatically increased the average life duration. The public health advancements that lowered newborn mortality, raised the likelihood that children would survive childhood, and prevented infection and communicable disease were the most significant. Currently, the average lifespan in the United States is around 80 years, while some people live significantly longer.

Scientists are researching persons in their 90s (known as nonagenarians) and 100s (known as centenarians, including supercentenarians, ages 110+), to see what factors contribute to their long lives. They discovered that people that live a long life differ greatly from one another in terms of occupation, money, and education. The differences they do have, however, are a reflection of their lifestyles; many are stress-tolerant, nonsmokers, and do not have obesity. Moreover, most are female. These older persons are less prone than their counterparts of the same age to develop age-related chronic diseases, such as high blood pressure, heart disease, cancer, and diabetes, as a result of their healthy lifestyle choices.

First-degree relatives are those who have a first-degree relative with a long-lived person. These persons are more likely to live longer and in better health than their peers. At age 70, the age-related illnesses that are prevalent in older persons are less likely to affect people whose parents are centenarians. The siblings of centenarians frequently enjoy long lives, and if they do develop age-related illnesses (such high blood pressure, heart disease, cancer, or type 2 diabetes), these illnesses manifest later than they do in the general population. The tendency for longer lifespans to run in families raises the possibility that shared genetics, lifestyle choices or both have a significant impact on longevity.

Genes associated with long life are now being studied. About 25% of the diversity in human life expectancy is thought to be genetically determined, however it is unclear which genes and how they affect longevity. The APOE, FOXO3, and CETP genes have a few common changes (referred to as polymorphisms) related with extended life lengths, although they are not present in all people with remarkable longevity. It's possible that several different genes, some of which have undiscovered variations, work together to promote long life.

The same gene variations that raise disease risk in humans with ordinary life spans have been found in supercentenarians through whole genome sequencing research. But there are other additional newly discovered gene variants in the supercentenarians that might favor lifespan. For the first seven or eight decades of life, lifestyle is thought to be a more important factor in determining health and lifespan than heredity. Some people can achieve a healthy old age with nutritious eating, moderate alcohol use, quitting smoking, and regular exercise; genetics then appear to play an increasingly significant part in maintaining individuals' health as they age into their eighties and beyond. Many nonagenarians and centenarians are able to live on their own and stay healthy well into their latter years of life.

Some of the gene variations that support a long life are connected to the fundamental upkeep and operation of the body's cells. These biological processes include DNA repair, upkeep of the telomeres at the ends of chromosomes, and defense of cells against injury by unstable oxygen-containing molecules (free radicals). The risk of heart disease (the leading cause of mortality in older adults), stroke, and insulin resistance is considerably decreased by other genes linked to blood fat (lipid) levels, inflammation, and the cardiovascular and immune systems.

The interaction of genetic and environmental factors is assumed to play a significant role in determining a person's lifespan. However, according to twin studies, just 20 to 30 percent of an individual's likelihood of living to age 85 may be attributed to genetics.

Unquestionably, one's lifestyle choices, particularly those related to nutrition, exercise, and smoking, affect both how long one will live and how gracefully they age. Seventh-Day Adventists have a well-documented average life expectancy of 88 years, which is around eight years longer than the typical American, according to studies, and their religion actively promotes activities that support good aging. Most Adventists engage in regular physical activity, follow a vegetarian diet, and abstain from smoking and alcohol.

However, a quick look at your family tree may reveal whether you have a hereditary propensity for longevity. According to research, there is a strong genetic component to extraordinary longevity (EL), which is defined as lasting one to three decades longer than the average U.S. life expectancy of about 80 years. In a press conference on Wednesday, Perls stated, "That...has always made us believe that genetics is playing a very important role in this wonderful trait."

There are at least two significant ways that genetic variables might influence how long someone lives: Other gene variants may give illness resistance, hence boosting lifespan. An individual may inherit specific genetic variations that predispose him or her to disease and reduce longevity.
The researchers examined the DNA of more than 800 people ranging in age from 95 to 119 and compared it to DNA from random controls in order to better understand the genetic factors influencing longevity. Specific genetic variants, or SNPs (single-nucleotide polymorphisms), were found to be connected to the longevity group by the genome-wide investigation.

The scientists then created a genetic model with 150 SNPs in order to calculate a person's propensity towards EL. With 77 percent accuracy, their model accurately predicted remarkable longevity in a distinct group of centenarians (those who live to be 100 years old). This proves that complex combinations of genetic variations are highly linked to EL.

Surprisingly, the researchers discovered that roughly 15% of the controls also have the gene signature linked to lifespan. This shows that far more people than previously believed had the genetic capacity to live into old life. Sebastiani stated, "We know a great deal about the human genome, but we also know that there is a great deal that remains to be discovered." Although essential to EL, genetics is not the main factor. Therefore, he added, "There may be more elements, such as the environment or different lifestyles, that help people live longer and healthier lives.

Role of lifestyle Factors in Longevity

Proverbs and adages on the value of good health have been used throughout history. Many stress the connection between good health and happiness, as well as the chance to lead a purposeful life.

The Japan Collaborate Cohort (JACC) Study group at Osaka University examined the effects of altering lifestyle behaviors on life expectancy beginning in middle age in a study published this month in Age and Ageing. The study's findings showed that adopting five or more healthy living practices extended life expectancy for all people, even those with chronic diseases and those over 80.

Social factors like
- Socioeconomic level,
- Governmental policies like assisted access to healthcare,
- Personal choices like nutrition and exercise all affect how long people live.

The purpose of the questionnaire was to gather more information about the variables that affect the risk of dying from cardiovascular disease and cancer. As a result, it had questions regarding body mass index, diet, exercise, and alcohol and cigarette use. Each healthy habit received points, and the effect of changing these lifestyle behaviors on expected lifespan was calculated.

By the end of the study in December 2009, 8,966 people had passed away. Dr. Ryoto Sakaniwa, the study's principal author, said. "The outcomes were pretty obvious. For both men and women, a higher percentage of modified healthy behaviors was strongly linked to long life. For healthy 40-year-olds, the lifetime gains were greatest for decreasing alcohol consumption, quitting smoking, losing weight, and getting more sleep, which added up to 6 years of life.

Even those who were older (80 years or more), had one or more serious comorbid conditions including cancer, cardiovascular disease, hypertension, diabetes, or kidney disease, or were at any period of life after middle age, this effect was noticeable.

The discovery that lifestyle changes can enhance health despite chronic illnesses and advanced age is encouraging, especially in light of the rising prevalence of chronic illnesses and longer life expectancies. The results of this study will help shape public health strategies, policies, and healthcare environments in the future that collaborate with patients to encourage healthy lifestyle choices.

We all want to live long and healthy lives as humans. While our lifespan is partly determined by our genes, there are several lifestyle choices that can help increase it. In this post, we'll talk about how lifestyle affects longevity and examine the various behaviors and decisions that might lead to longer, better lives.

Diet is the first aspect of lifestyle that can shorten our lifespan. Our health and lifespan can be significantly impacted by the foods we eat. A lower risk of chronic diseases like heart disease, cancer, and diabetes has been linked to a diet high in fruits, vegetables, whole grains, and lean meats. However, consuming a lot of processed meals, trans fats, and saturated fats and sugary drinks can increase the risk of diseases and shorten our lifespan.

Exercise on a regular basis is yet another essential lifestyle choice that may affect our longevity. It has been demonstrated that participating in physical activity for at least 30 minutes a day lowers the chance of developing chronic diseases and enhances general health. In addition to maintaining a healthy weight, exercise can help you live a long and healthy life.

Two lifestyle choices that can be harmful to our health and longevity are smoking and drinking too much alcohol. Smoking has been connected to a number of cancers, heart disease, and respiratory conditions, and it is the greatest cause of preventable deaths in the world. Similar to how excessive alcohol intake can result in cancer, liver damage, and other health issues. We can live longer, healthier lives by limiting or avoiding certain habits. Another element that may shorten our lifespan is stress. Heart disease, depression, and other health issues have all been associated with chronic stress. Spending time in nature or participating in stress-relieving exercises like yoga or meditation can help you manage stress and enhance your general wellbeing.

Last but not least, longevity has also been associated with social support and a sense of purpose. Strong ties to friends and family can offer emotional support and lower the chance of developing depression and other mental health problems. A longer and better life can also result from discovering your mission in life.

In conclusion, lifestyle choices have a big impact on how long we live. Developing healthy habits, such as eating well, exercising frequently, abstaining from vices, and managing stress,and maintaining social connections can help us live longer, healthier lives. By making these lifestyle changes, we can take control of our health and increase our chances of living a long and fulfilling life.

CHAPTER 2 : NUTRITION AND LONGEVITY

The importance of healthy diet for longevity

It is impossible to exaggerate the value of a nutritious diet for extending life. Our daily health and wellbeing are impacted by the foods we eat, but they can also shorten our lives. According to research, eating a diet rich in fruits, vegetables, whole grains, and lean proteins can help prevent chronic illnesses like diabetes, cancer, and diseases like heart disease that are major causes of early mortality. On the other hand, a diet rich in trans and saturated fats, processed foods, and sweetened beverages can raise our risk of developing chronic illnesses and reduce our life expectancy. The vital role that a healthy diet plays in promoting longevity, the specific minerals and foods that can support a long and healthy life, and helpful advice for adopting a healthy diet into your daily life are all covered in this Chapter.

Here are some of the Benefits of a healthy diet for Longevity.

- Reduced risk of chronic illnesses: A diet high in fruits, vegetables, whole grains, and lean proteins can aid in the prevention of chronic illnesses including diabetes, cancer, and heart disease, which are important causes of early mortality. These foods are rich in essential nutrients and anti-inflammatory compounds that can shield our cells from harm and inflammation, lowering the risk of illness.
- Reduced risk of heart disease, stroke, and other cardiovascular issues: Eating a nutritious diet can also reduce one's risk of developing heart disease, stroke, and other cardiovascular issues. This is because a nutritious diet can aid in reducing inflammation, blood pressure, and cholesterol levels, all of which are risk factors for heart disease.
- Better weight management: Another significant component in enhancing longevity is maintaining a healthy weight. By supplying the minerals and energy we require without adding extra calories, a nutritious diet can assist us in achieving and maintaining a healthy weight. Because obesity is a significant risk factor for many chronic diseases, this is crucial.

- Healthy eating can also aid in improving cognitive function and lowering the risk of dementia and Alzheimer's disease. Antioxidants and omega-3 fatty acids, which are nutrients present in fruits, vegetables, and whole grains, have been demonstrated to enhance brain health and function.
- Finally, a healthy diet can enhance our general quality of life by lowering our chance of developing depression, anxiety, and other mental health issues. It can also give us the vitality and vigor we require to fully appreciate life.
- A nutritious diet is essential for boosting lifespan as well as general health and wellbeing, to sum up. We can lower our chance of developing chronic illnesses, improve heart health, maintain a healthy weight, enhance cognitive function, and live longer by consuming nutrient-dense meals instead of processed and unhealthy alternatives.

The best foods for Longevity

The food we consume has the power to either benefit or hurt us. Our dependence on processed foods deprives us of enough nutrition and contributes to diseases like obesity, cardiovascular disease, and type 2 diabetes. It doesn't have to be this way; instead, we should eat things that give us energy, lower our chance of being sick, and let us keep a healthy weight. We need to nourish our bodies with nutrient-dense foods if we want to live longer and be healthy. Our health and vigor can be recovered with natural plant foods.

A] Cruciferous Plants

These are superfood vegetables with the rare capacity to alter human hormones, stimulate the body's inherent cleansing process, and stop the development of malignant cells. To release their potent anti-cancer qualities, cruciferous vegetables should be chewed thoroughly or consumed shredded, diced, juiced, or mixed. Sulforaphane, a phytochemical found in crucifers, has been discovered to shield blood vessel walls from inflammatory signals, which can cause heart disease. The foods that are highest in nutrients are cruciferous veggies. Consume a variety of foods every day, both raw and cooked. Try some broccoli, cauliflower, Brussels sprouts, kale, or cabbage.

B] Salad Greens

Raw, cruciferous leafy green vegetables have less than 100 calories per pound, making them an excellent diet for weight management. In scientific studies, women who started meals with a large salad consumed fewer calories overall, and larger salads did so more effectively than smaller ones. Increased consumption of salads, leafy greens, or raw vegetables is linked to lower risk of heart attack, stroke, diabetes, and a number of malignancies in addition to maintaining a healthy weight. In addition to the necessary B vitamin folate, leafy greens are also a good source of the carotenoids lutein and zeaxanthin, which shield the eyes from harmful light. Try spinach, kale, mustard greens, collard greens, or lettuce. To get the most health advantages from leafy greens, you need to absorb their fat-soluble phytochemicals, particularly their carotenoids, and to do that, you need fats. For this reason, your salad (or dressing) should always contain nuts and/or seeds.

C] Nuts

Nuts are an essential part of an anti-diabetes diet because they are a high-nutrient source of beneficial fats, plant protein, fiber, antioxidants, phytosterols, and minerals. They are also a low-glycemic food that helps lower the glycemic load of an entire meal. Consuming nuts is linked to lower body weight despite their high calorie content, possibly as a result of the heart-healthy components' ability to suppress appetite. Regular nut consumption lowers cholesterol and is associated with a 35% lower risk of heart disease. Your next salad can be topped with chopped walnuts or sliced almonds, or you can make a creamy salad dressing with some raw cashews.

D] **Seeds**
Although seeds include more protein and more trace minerals than nuts, their nutritional profile is remarkably comparable to that of nuts in that both contain beneficial fats, minerals, and antioxidants. Hemp, chia, and flax seeds are full of omega-3 fatty acids. Phytoestrogens that prevent breast cancer, lignans, are also abundant in flax, chia, and sesame seeds. Pumpkin seeds are particularly high in zinc, whereas sesame seeds are high in calcium and vitamin E. Nuts and seeds should be consumed raw or very gently roasted for the greatest nutritional benefit. To your morning smoothie or oatmeal, try adding flax or chia seeds.

E] **Berries**
These fruits are a great source of heart-healthy antioxidants. Studies showing reductions in blood pressure, oxidative stress indicators, total and LDL cholesterol in those who consumed blueberries or strawberries on a daily basis for several weeks. Berries are a great brain food and have anti-cancer qualities as well. There is proof that eating berries may help delay the effects of aging on the brain. Choose tried-and-true fruits like strawberries or blueberries instead, or try something novel like goji berries.

F] **Pomegranate**
The pomegranate is a special fruit with tiny, crisp, juicy arils that have a delicious blend of sweet and sour flavors. Punicalagin, the most prevalent and distinctive phytochemical of pomegranates, is responsible for more than half of the antioxidant activity of pomegranate juice. The phytochemicals in pomegranates have a number of anti-cancer, heart-protective, and brain-healthy effects. A study of individuals with severe carotid artery blockages who drank one ounce of pomegranate juice every day for a year discovered a 30% reduction in atherosclerotic plaque; in the control group, atherosclerotic plaque grew by 9%. This study is noteworthy because it involved patients who had severe carotid artery blockages. In a different research of senior citizens, those who drank pomegranate juice every day for 28 days outperformed those who drank a placebo drink on a memory test.Observer advice: To remove the fruit's edible arils, score it about a half-inch deep on the diameter, twist to

separate it into two pieces, and then pound the back of each piece with the back of a heavy spoon.

G] **Beans**
Consuming beans and other legumes on a regular basis can help control your blood sugar, curb your appetite, and prevent colon cancer. Beans are the most nutrient-dense source of starch, and because of their slow digestion, which reduces blood glucose spikes after meals and encourages satiety, they are also an effective weight-loss and anti-diabetes diet. They also have a lot of soluble fiber, which lowers cholesterol, and resistant starch, which is transformed into short-chain fatty acids by intestinal bacteria and prevents colon cancer. It has been discovered that eating beans, peas, or lentils twice a week reduces the risk of colon cancer by 50%. Consuming legumes significantly reduces the risk of developing other malignancies as well.

H] **Mushrooms**
Consuming beans and other legumes on a regular basis can help control your blood sugar, curb your appetite, and prevent colon cancer. Beans are the most nutrient-dense source of starch, and because of their slow digestion, which reduces blood glucose spikes after meals and encourages satiety, they are also an effective weight-loss and anti-diabetes diet. They also have a lot of soluble fiber, which lowers cholesterol, and resistant starch, which is transformed into short-chain fatty acids by intestinal bacteria and prevents colon cancer. It has been discovered that eating beans, peas, or lentils twice a week reduces the risk of colon cancer by 50%. Consuming legumes significantly reduces the risk of developing other malignancies as well. Try them all and pick your favorites. Red beans, black beans, chickpeas, lentils, and split peas are all delicious.

I] **Onions and Garlic**
Onions, a member of the allium family of plants, have positive effects on the cardiovascular and immunological systems as well as having anti-diabetic and anti-cancer properties. Prostate and stomach cancer risk are inversely correlated with allium vegetable diet. These vegetables are

well-known for their organosulfur compounds, which work to detoxify carcinogens, slow cancer cell proliferation, and prevent angiogenesis, all of which contribute to the prevention of cancer. When these substances are chewed, crushed, or chopped, these components are released. Additionally, onions are rich in flavonoid antioxidants, which are known to have anti-inflammatory properties and may help prevent cancer. Try leeks, chives, shallots, and scallions as alternatives to garlic and yellow onions.

J] **Tomatoes**

An abundance of health-promoting nutrients can be found in tomatoes – lycopene, vitamins C and E, beta-carotene and flavanol antioxidants, to name but a few. Lycopene in particular protects against prostate cancer, UV skin damage and cardiovascular disease. About 85 percent of the lycopene in American diets is derived from tomatoes. Lycopene is more absorbable when tomatoes are cooked – one cup of tomato sauce has 10 times the lycopene as one cup of raw, chopped tomatoes. Also keep in mind that carotenoids, like lycopene, are best absorbed when accompanied by healthy fats, so enjoy your tomatoes in a salad with nuts or a nut-based dressing for extra nutritional punch. Tip: buy diced and crushed tomatoes in glass jars, not cans, to avoid the endocrine disruptor BPA in can liners.

Role of Supplements in Longevity

It's crucial to keep in mind that supplements are just that: additional. The best method to receive the vitamins, minerals, and antioxidants you require is through a healthy, nutritious diet, however supplements are useful for giving you a little boost when you are deficient in particular nutrients.

According to Kara Burnstine, RD, a nutrition expert at Pritikin Longevity Center, "Supplements will never give you what actual, real food will," "They merely assist you. They are not intended to replace food.
Burnstine acknowledges that relying only on food for sustenance can have drawbacks and that supplements can sometimes be helpful.
"It would be wonderful if we all ate all of our fruits, vegetables, whole grains, and lean proteins and got everything that we needed from the food supply, but unfortunately, our food supply is sometimes not the highest quality either," she says. Therefore, even though we can be doing a lot of nice things, we might not be getting all the nutrients from our food.
According to her, this shortfall may worsen as you age.
"Since we are machines, as we age, things that formerly operated well begin to fail. We may then need to use supplements more frequently at that point.

Not everyone should use every vitamin. Before beginning any supplement, you should always speak with your doctor to make sure it won't conflict with any medications you're already taking or put you at risk for other issues. However, Burnstine suggests the following for the majority of those nearing or in their golden years:

A] Calcium for strong bones
You can benefit from calcium in many ways. It aids in blood clotting, promotes muscle contraction, and maintains healthy neuron and heart rhythms. Additionally, it helps to maintain strong bones. Your body draws calcium from your bones to maintain proper function when you don't consume enough of it. You can replace this calcium and maintain strong bones by consuming calcium on a daily basis.
Your daily calcium requirement increases once you become 50. Before then, 1,200 milligrams a day will suffice, but once you reach 50, you need increase to 1,500 milligrams a day. The disease osteoporosis poses the greatest threat to women who have experienced menopause.
According to Burnstine, a calcium supplement is an excellent choice if you are aware that you are not consuming at least two servings from a calcium source each day. The supplement, however, is just one element of the

jigsaw.In addition to the calcium pill, she advises doing resistance exercise, which protects bones more than anything else, and consuming at least two meals of dairy products or a lot of green leafy vegetables.

B] Vitamin D for strong bones and immunity
Speaking of strong bones, vitamin D is required for your body to absorb calcium. Vitamin D also has neuroprotective, anti-inflammatory, and antioxidant effects. It supports the work of the brain cells, muscles, and immune system.
You must obtain vitamin D from external sources because your body cannot produce it. Food, the sun, or supplements are a few examples. Your daily need is 600 IU before the age of 70. It rises to 800 IU after 70. Your body might require a boost as you age in order to accomplish these goals.

C] **Probiotics for Gut health**
Recent research suggests that probiotic supplements may help prevent age-related changes in gut microbiota, enhancing immune function and supporting healthy digestion as you age. Probiotics are the "good" bacteria that dwell in your digestive system and help keep "bad" bacteria in check.
"We know that if our gut health is good, everything else follows, in terms of inflammation, brain fog, weight loss, sleep, and depression," claims Burnstine. "Our gut is connected to almost everything,"
It's better to obtain probiotics through the foods you eat, just like with other nutrients. Fermented foods including yogurt, kefir, kombucha, chilled sauerkraut, kimchi, tempeh, and miso might help you stock up on them. A supplement, though, is not a bad idea. Although some supplements contain up to 50 billion colony-forming units (CFUs), Burnstine claims that your body only absorbs 20% to 30% of that quantity.

D] **Magnesium for Mood**
Magnesium is linked to enzymatic processes, immunological function, and it helps to reduce inflammation. It also plays a significant role in mood stability. As you become older, your magnesium levels decrease, increasing your risk of mental health issues.According to Burnstine, those with low magnesium levels are more likely to experience depression. Chronically

low levels can also raise your risk for heart disease, type 2 diabetes, high blood pressure, and osteoporosis.

Everyone over the age of 30 needs 320–420 milligrams of magnesium per day, but not all magnesium supplements are created equal, according to Burnstine.

You may, for instance, take magnesium carbonate, but you could also take magnesium glycinate, which is a little softer on the stomach, advises the expert. "The way it's put together results in a variety of responses," Discuss the ideal magnesium formulation for you with your doctor.

E] **A Multivitamin to cover all bases**
While not a cure-all, a daily multivitamin can improve your overall nutritional status. According to Burnstine, it won't hurt if nothing else.

A multivitamin is kind of like an insurance policy, I usually say, she continues. "At any age, I would advise taking a general multivitamin." Although most brands are similar, search for the USP sign for assurance. This seal of approval designates products whose quality is consistent and which contain the precise components in the potency and quantity specified on the label.

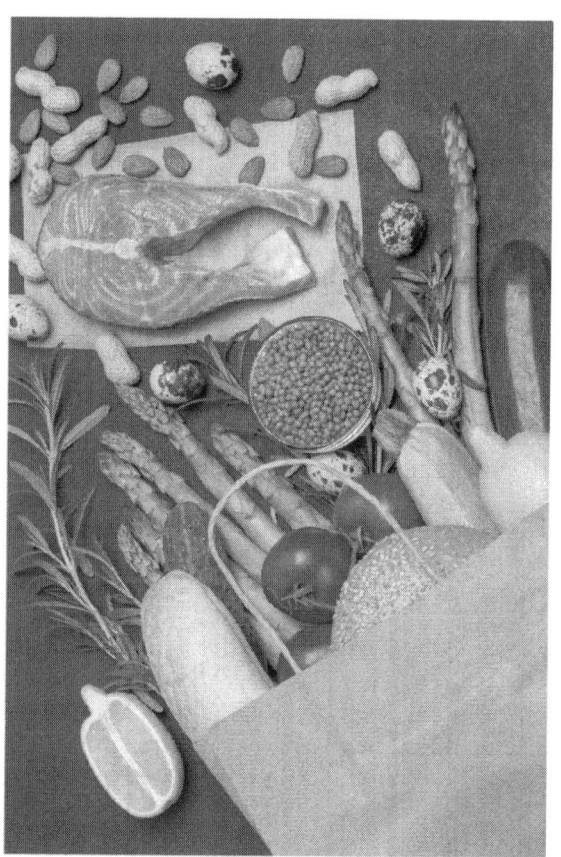

CHAPTER 3: EXERCISE AND LONGEVITY

The Benefits of Exercise for Longevity

The importance of exercise in maintaining a healthy lifestyle has long been acknowledged, and its advantages extend beyond mere physical wellbeing. Regular physical activity has often been proved to considerably increase a person's longevity and general quality of life. Exercise can enhance cognitive performance, mental health, and general wellbeing in addition to preventing chronic diseases including heart disease, diabetes, and some types of cancer. Exercise has been related to a longer life expectancy, allowing people to live longer, healthier, and more active lives in addition to these physical and mental advantages. Exercise has established itself as a pillar of good living and longevity, which is not surprising given the rising emphasis on preventative health and wellbeing.

No matter your age, staying active is crucial. Both your body and mind benefit from exercise.

How does that happen? And how can you implement it into your life most effectively?

The Benefits of Exercise
- Lower your blood pressure
- Manage stress and improve your mood
- Ease symptoms of anxiety and depression
- Lower your chances of heart disease
- Manage chronic conditions like arthritis or diabetes by helping with things like stamina, joint swelling, pain, and muscle strength
- Help with your balance, so you're less likely to fall and break bones

Types of Exercise that promote Longevity

You can feel a little intimidated by exercising as you age. You might believe that you need to join a gym or that you risk injuring yourself. Or perhaps you are unsure of the exercises you ought to perform.

Not where or how you start being active matters; just start moving.
The weekly recommended amount for active people in good health is 150 minutes of heart- and blood-pumping activity. Yes, with exercise classes you can do that. But vigorous walking is another way to obtain it.
Additionally, it's crucial to perform exercises that train all of your major muscles at least twice a week. To help with your range of motion, attempt to practice flexibility exercises two or three days a week as well.
Although 150 minutes may seem lengthy, you don't have to complete it in lengthy segments. You can sweep the porch for 10 minutes or go for a 10-minute walk around the neighborhood. All of it adds up.
If you have the energy, you can increase your weekly exercise time to at least 300 minutes for even greater health advantages.

But a straightforward objective is to make an effort to engage in moderate-intensity exercise for 30 minutes most days. Some weeks you might be able to achieve it, other weeks maybe not. Keep in mind that it's a goal, not a rule. Go with what suits you.

How to Move Forward
Exercise and physical activity are two methods to move.
Exercise is any organized exercise, such as spinning, tai chi, aerobics, or swimming. The way you "sneak" movement into your day is through physical activity, such as gardening or dog walking. You'll live longer and be healthier if you incorporate both into your regimen. But before becoming dramatically more active, always consult your doctor.

You don't need expensive clothing or accessories. You can start things out in a less formal manner by:

- Go for a quick stroll or jog.
- Use a bicycle
- Sweep the lawn or operate a lawn mower.
- Broom or dust
- Take up tennis
- Climb and descend stairs

- Deliver groceries

In just a few weeks, you should begin to feel stronger and more energetic. Then, if you feel up to it, you can visit a gym or community center to participate in strength-training activities, dance courses, or water aerobics.

Tips for staying Active

Exercise frequently: Exercise frequently is necessary to maintain both healthy physical and mental health. In addition to enhancing flexibility, balance, and coordination and lowering the risk of chronic diseases, it can also improve mood and cognitive performance. On most days of the week, try to get in at least 30 minutes of moderate-intensity activity, such as brisk walking, cycling, or swimming.

Maintain your social networks: Social networks are crucial for mental and emotional health. Strong interpersonal ties with one's family, friends, and community can ease stress, improve mood, and give one a feeling of purpose and belonging.

Continue your education: Continuing your education can keep your mind busy and bright. Think about enrolling in a course, joining a reading club, or taking up a brand-new activity.

Consume a healthy, balanced diet: Chronic diseases can be avoided and good health can be maintained with a healthy diet. Choose a wide range of nutrient-dense foods, such as fresh produce, whole grains, lean proteins, and healthy fats.

Get enough sleep: Sleep is essential for emotional, cognitive, and physical health. Establish a regular sleep schedule and aim for 7-8 hours of sleep each night.

Practice relaxation methods: Relaxation methods, such as yoga, deep breathing exercises, and meditation, can assist to lower tension and encourage relaxation. Think about implementing these routines into your day.

Keep moving all day long: In addition to regular exercise, strive to keep moving all day long by incorporating movement into your everyday routine. While watching TV, take frequent breaks to stretch or take a stroll, stand up and get some exercise during commercials, and use the stairs rather than the elevator.

Recall that maintaining good physical health, mental wellbeing, and overall quality of life in old age requires continued physical activity. You may maintain your health, activity level, and engagement far into your golden years by adopting these suggestions into your daily routine.

CHAPTER 4: SLEEP AND LONGEVITY

The Importance of Sleep for Longevity

Living healthier, longer lives has been a primary, though elusive, lifelong aim for many people. Recent technological breakthroughs and ground-breaking scientific discoveries have thrown light on this issue. One of the greatest accomplishments of the 20th century was the enormous increase in the average life expectancy around the world. The life expectancy at birth increased from 31 years in 1900 to around 73 years in 2021.

Helping individuals age successfully is now a top concern in healthcare. Disease prevention and quality of life will both benefit from slowing down or even stopping the aging process. Scientists are looking into habits that can be used to increase future generations' life expectancy well over 100, rather than trying to create a miraculous cure, and they may have the solution.

Let's talk about the one activity we all engage in that already consumes a third of our lives: sleeping. This shouldn't be a shock to anyone. Numerous vital physiological processes occur during sleep, however they are by no means limited to:

Immunity
metabolic process
hormonal (endocrine) activity
Cognition
Thermoregulation
Getting rid of waste in the brain

Now, according to scientists, getting enough, regular, and high-quality sleep may be the key to raising the world's average life expectancy. According to research, people who are able to survive to a very late age—the uncommon centenarians who reach the age of 100—have usually healthy sleep patterns throughout their lives. However, lack of sleep can hasten the aging process because it has an impact on almost all bodily physiological processes. Prior to delving into the data analyzing the connection between sleep and longevity, it's critical to comprehend how sleep varies over the course of a person's lifespan.

Our ability to sleep worsens with aging. In actuality, sleep undergoes significant modification over time. So much so that our sleep's duration and quality can be utilized as a window through which to see how quickly our brains are aging. You can see a "hypnogram" (a graphic intended to assist visualize sleep and its various stages) below. The top graphic shows that young adults often go through a rhythmic and organized number of stages of sleep at night. The night begins with a large amount of deep sleep (represented by NREM-3 and NREM-4), then REM sleep increases.
This trend changes in older persons, who also experience a large increase in sleep fragmentation. There is less time spent in REM and deep sleep, and there is more time spent awake throughout the night.

Additionally, more than simply the length or frequency of these sleep stages are disturbed. The quality of the various sleep stages deteriorates. As we get older, the slow waves that are present during deep sleep and are in charge of numerous crucial processes become less powerful and dense. Sleep spindles, which are a defining feature of NREM sleep, slow down and become less frequent in older people. In summary, as we become older, the brain's capacity to produce normal electrical activity connected to sleep reduces.
But this isn't how things usually work. Older folks don't suddenly need less sleep than they did; they can't produce the same amount of sleep that's still necessary. There are similarities between this and how scientists are starting to see aging. According to some scientists, it's time to classify aging as a disease that we should strive to cure, rather than as a natural consequence of life.

Quantity of Sleep and Lifespan
We really begin to see the possible correlations between inadequate sleep and mortality when we examine data from prospective cohort studies, or long-term studies following populations across time.
Consider the Finnish Twin Study from the first half of the 1980s. In this investigation, sleep quality and hypnotic usage were tracked in identical twins over the course of their lifetime. These results were connected with all-cause mortality, also known as death from any cause. Before going into the results, it's crucial to emphasize that these studies are simply estimating connections and cannot determine the exact reason why sleep may affect longevity. These research should also be qualified by some significant cautions.

Quantity of Sleep and Lifespan
We really begin to see the possible correlations between inadequate sleep and mortality when we examine data from prospective cohort studies, or long-term studies following populations across time.
Consider the Finnish Twin Study from the first half of the 1980s. In this investigation, sleep quality and hypnotic usage were tracked in identical twins over the course of their lifetime. These results were connected with all-cause mortality, also known as death from any cause. Before going into the results, it's crucial to emphasize that these studies are simply estimating connections and cannot determine the exact reason why sleep may affect longevity. These research should also be qualified by some significant cautions.
These include relying excessively on self-reported sleep measurements and failing to consider personal sleep preferences and requirements. Having said that, what they discovered was unexpected.
First, a twofold increase in the chance of dying from any cause was linked to adult use of hypnotics and/or tranquilizers on a regular basis. Next, despite finding an increased risk of death from all causes in short sleepers—those who get less than 7 hours of sleep each night—the researchers also discovered similar increases in those who get more than 9 hours of sleep. When we examine individuals in other groups as well as the overall population, we notice comparable trends. In another study,

all-cause mortality was linked to both getting less than 7 hours of sleep per night and getting more than 9 hours.

Other research indicates a connection between lengthy and short sleep durations and the risk of stroke. Stroke risk is also markedly increased by sleep disorders like obstructive sleep apnea, restless legs syndrome, and insomnia. Long sleepers also seem to be more susceptible to other illnesses, like coronary heart disease, which is the main cause of mortality in the US.

These findings imply that there may be a "Goldilocks zone" for the amount of time one should sleep, beyond which the risk of illness development and even shortening life span increases.

To fully comprehend why getting more sleep isn't always beneficial, more study is necessary. Do those who sleep a lot spend the majority of the night in lighter stages of sleep, with little to no REM or deep sleep? Are there any additional conditions that long sleepers have that are causing them to live shorter lives? There is still no clear solution to these queries.

Sleep, Illness, and Lifespan

The evidence on brief sleep duration and longevity is, in general, better explained. For instance, a recent study discovered a higher risk of dementia in people who slept fewer than 6 hours every night around middle age. In instance, compared to persistent normal sleep length, persistent short sleep duration at ages 50, 60, and 70 was likewise linked to a 30% increased risk of dementia, regardless of other possibly confounding factors.

Impaired glucose metabolism, or the mechanism that makes sure that living cells always have an energy source, is also linked to both poor sleep quality and short sleep duration. The metabolism of glucose is significantly affected after 5 nights of barely 4 hours of sleep. The effects of slow-wave sleep deprivation are likewise similar, underlining the value of deep sleep for healthy bodily processes. When considered collectively, the effects of sleep loss on glucose metabolism may encourage the onset of obesity, diabetes, and other endocrine/hormonal disorders, further lowering quality of life and shortening lifespan.

The Best Sleeping Patterns and Longevity

What then, are the best sleep features of the long-lived? In one study, sleep habits were examined between "the oldest of old individuals" (those between 85 and 105 years old) and younger and older adults (60 to 70 years old). In contrast to older persons, those who lived longer had regular and reliable sleep-wake schedules and maintained appropriate amounts of slow-wave (deep) sleep, the researchers discovered.

Another study looked at the relationship between sleep habits and health in long-lived families. Despite being more likely to exhibit risk sleep habits (such as oversleeping and napping), the researchers discovered that centenarians were protected from age-related variables. This finding raises the possibility that specific genes may be protective against the negative consequences of sleep disturbance.

Finally, Japanese researchers looked at the sleep habits and way of life of residents of Ogimi, a community known for its long life. People in the community who had "good sleep health" were more likely to take quick naps, to not fall asleep in the middle of the day, and to engage in regular exercise.

Sleep is undoubtedly a crucial component of good health and wellbeing. Inadequate sleep impacts practically every physiological function in the body and is linked to the onset and progression of disease. Optimal sleep may be the single most important pillar at resetting and rebuilding our body. By making sleep a non-negotiable priority and adhering to sleep hygiene advice. You may start to utilize the power of sleep.

How to Improve your Sleep Habits

- Maintain a consistent sleep schedule by attempting to go to bed and wake up at the same time each day, including on the weekends.

- Make sure your bedroom is dark, quiet, and cool to promote restful sleep.

- Make use of soft cushions and a firm mattress.
- Reduce your screen time before bed because the blue light that electronic devices emit can disrupt your sleep. At least an hour before going to bed, avoid using electronics.
- Take a warm bath, meditate, or engage in some yoga or deep breathing exercises to unwind before bed.
- Avoid caffeine, alcohol, and nicotine because these might induce sleep disruption and frequent awakenings.
- Exercise frequently; however, avoid exercising too close to bedtime since it may keep you awake. Exercise can enhance the quality of your sleep.
- Avoid eating a heavy dinner right before bed because it will make it uncomfortable and harder to fall asleep.
- Avoid taking too many naps throughout the day as this can interfere with your ability to sleep at night. If you must snooze, do so early in the day and make it brief.
- Reduce your stress levels because they can disturb your sleep. Learn how to control your stress levels by engaging in soothing activities, talking to a therapist, or practicing mindfulness.
- Get some exposure to the sun: Sunlight helps to control your circadian cycle, which is necessary for a restful night's sleep. Get outside during the day or, if you live somewhere with little natural light, think about buying a light treatment lamp.

CHAPTER 5: STRESS MANAGEMENT AND LONGEVITY

Life will always involve some level of stress. Whether it's brought on by relationships, the workplace, or other everyday difficulties, it happens to everyone of us occasionally. Chronic stress, however, can have negative effects on our physical and mental health, as well as a shorter lifespan. As a result, learning efficient stress management skills is crucial for promoting longevity and general wellbeing.

The Effects of Stress on Health

Stress is a typical reaction to difficult circumstances, and it has certain positive effects in moderation. It can enhance our performance and keep us alert and focused. However, persistent stress can be detrimental to our health.

Chronic stress can trigger an overactive stress response that increases the risk of heart disease, stroke, and other chronic illnesses as well as inflammation and high blood pressure. Additionally, it may weaken our immune systems, leaving us more vulnerable to illnesses and infections. Chronic stress can also exacerbate mental health issues like depression and anxiety.

Stress Management Techniques

We may fortunately lessen stress and its detrimental effects on our health by using appropriate stress management practices. The following methods have been shown to increase longevity and wellbeing:

- The practice of mindfulness meditation can significantly lower stress and anxiety. It entails concentrating on the present and embracing it without criticism. According to studies, practicing mindfulness meditation can lower blood pressure, lessen stress, and enhance general wellbeing.

- Exercise: Regular exercise has a variety of advantages for both physical and mental health. It can aid in stress reduction, mood enhancement, and longevity promotion. Endorphins are naturally occurring substances that improve mood, and exercise can stimulate endorphin production.

- Social Support: A strong social support system can help us manage stress and lengthen our lives. A sense of belonging can be created and loneliness and isolation can be lessened by spending time with friends and loved ones.
- Deep breathing, gradual muscle relaxation, and visualization are all examples of relaxation techniques that can help people unwind and reduce stress. These methods are simple to learn and may be used anywhere.
- Time management: By enabling us to prioritize work and prevent feeling overloaded, effective time management can help us feel less stressed. We can feel more in control of our time and less stressed and anxious by planning and arranging our responsibilities.

Conclusion

The effects of persistent stress on our health and wellness can be severe. However, there are practical stress-reduction strategies that might help us lessen anxiety and increase longevity. Effective stress management strategies include mindfulness meditation, physical activity, social support, relaxation techniques, and time management. By utilizing these strategies into our daily lives, we can reduce stress and enjoy a longer healthier life.

CHAPTER 6: SOCIAL CONNECTIONS AND LONGEVITY

The Role of Social Connections in Longevity

Studies have shown that having strong social links can result in a longer, healthier life. Social connections play a significant part in our health and wellness. In this post, we'll look at the numerous ways that social support can affect our health as well as the part it plays in lifespan.

Social Connections' Effect on Health

Numerous studies have demonstrated that social relationships can significantly affect our health and happiness. A Harvard School of Public Health study, for instance, discovered that people with strong social links had a 50% higher risk of living longer than those with weak social ties. According to a different study published in the Journal of Health and Social Behavior, people with larger social networks had lower risk of mortality. Our social ties can have a variety of effects on our health. Stress reduction is one of the most important methods. Stress and anxiety can be reduced with the aid of social support, which may improve our physical health. Social ties can also encourage us to exercise, eat healthily, and abstain from bad habits, which can all help us maintain a healthy lifestyle.

Relationships with Others and Mental Health

Our mental health can be significantly impacted by our social interactions as well. Mental health issues like sadness and anxiety can arise as a result of loneliness and social isolation. On the other hand, having healthy social ties can lift our spirits and give us a sense of purpose and belonging.

Additionally, social connections might support us in overcoming challenging life circumstances. The emotional support and practical help we require to overcome obstacles and keep a good attitude on life can be obtained by having a support system in place.

The Value of Retaining Social Relationships

Our social ties may deteriorate as we age for a variety of reasons, including retirement, the death of friends and relatives, and physical constraints. However, since they can have a considerable impact on our health and wellbeing, it's crucial to make an effort to keep up social ties.
Joining social clubs, giving back to the community, and attending events are just a few options for keeping up social ties. Furthermore, technology has made staying connected with family and friends simpler than ever.

In summary, research indicates that social ties can significantly affect our longevity and that they play a critical role in our health and wellbeing. We can lessen stress, enhance our mental health, and uphold a healthy lifestyle by keeping solid social links and looking for social support. Making an intentional effort to preserve social relationships and stay in touch with those around us is crucial as we become older.

How to maintain connections as you age

- Our social networks may change as we get older owing to a variety of reasons, including retirement, the death of friends and family members, and physical constraints. To keep socially engaged as we age, however, is important for our health and wellness, and there are various methods to do so. We will look at some advice on preserving social connections as you become older in this book.

- Join clubs and social groups: Getting involved in social groups and clubs is a great method to network and maintain relationships. There are numerous possibilities, including book clubs, exercise programs, and hobby organizations. A wonderful method to meet people who share your interests and form new friendships is to join a group that is related to them.

- Volunteer: Another fantastic approach to maintain relationships with others and give back to your community is through volunteering. Additionally, volunteering can give us a sense of fulfillment and purpose, which is good for our mental health. Look for volunteer options that fit your hobbies or abilities, such as working at a nearby animal shelter or hospital.
- Take Part in Local Events: Participating in neighborhood gatherings like fairs, festivals, and fundraisers is a great way to network and stay involved in your neighborhood. These gatherings give people a chance to interact socially and build relationships while also promoting regional companies and nonprofits.

- Make use of technology: The ability to stay in touch with people, especially those who live far away, has never been simpler thanks to technology. We may communicate with friends and family and share information about our life on social media sites like Facebook and Instagram. Additionally, we can engage with people face-to-face even when we are not in the same geographical location thanks to video chat platforms like Zoom and Skype.
- Attend workshops or classes: It's a great opportunity to meet new people and gain new skills to take classes or attend seminars. Such as culinary lessons or art workshops, look for classes or workshops that are relevant to your hobbies. These kinds of classes provide students the chance to interact with others and make new friends while also learning new things.

- Be Active: Our physical and emotional health depend on staying active, and it's also a great way to maintain relationships with other people. It's a terrific way to meet new people and keep active at the same time to join a fitness class or workout group.

As a result, it is crucial for our health and welfare to maintain social relationships, and there are various methods to do so as we get older. Joining social groups and clubs, volunteering, taking part in local events, using technology, going to workshops or classes, and being active are all fantastic ways to stay in touch with others and keep a feeling of purpose and belonging. As we age, we can enhance our quality of life and lead happier, healthier, and more satisfying lives by making a conscious effort to stay connected with people.

The Benefits of Volunteering and giving back for longevity

Numerous advantages for both physical and mental health have been linked to volunteering and community service. In fact, research have shown a correlation between volunteering and a longer lifespan and a lower risk of developing chronic illnesses.

Being socially linked is one of the key advantages of volunteering. Numerous health issues, such as melancholy, anxiety, and cardiovascular disease, are significantly increased by social isolation. Volunteering gives people the chance to make new friends and develop social ties, which helps lessen feelings of isolation and loneliness.

Volunteering has been demonstrated to enhance mental health in addition to social connectedness. According to studies, those who volunteer report reduced levels of despair and anxiety and higher levels of happiness. Additionally, volunteering can provide people a sense of direction and meaning in life, which can make them feel more content and happy in their daily lives.

Additionally connected to advantages for one's physical health is volunteering. For instance, a study indicated that older persons who donated at least 200 hours annually had a decreased chance of getting hypertension than those who did not volunteer. This finding was reported in the Journal of Gerontology. There is evidence from further research that volunteering can lower your chance of developing heart disease, stroke, and dementia.

Volunteering can keep people active and engaged, which is one reason it might be good for physical health. Many volunteer jobs include physical labor, such as gardening, park cleanup, or participation in charity walks and runs. People can lower their chance of developing chronic diseases and preserve their general health and wellbeing by engaging in regular physical activity.

Finally, volunteering can give people the chance to develop new talents and obtain worthwhile experience. For people wishing to change careers or who are returning to the workforce after a period of unemployment, this can be very helpful. People who volunteer can improve their resumes, learn new skills, and form meaningful connections that could result in future employment chances.

In conclusion, volunteering and community service can have a variety of positive effects on one's physical and mental health. Volunteering can contribute to a person living a longer, healthier, and more meaningful life by encouraging social connectedness, creating a sense of purpose and meaning, and providing chances for physical activity and skill development.

VOLUNTEER TODAY

CHAPTER 7: ENVIRONMENTAL FACTORS AND LONGEVITY

How Environmental Factors Can Impact longevity

Genetics, dietary habits, and environmental circumstances are just a few of the many variables that might affect how long a person lives. Environmental influences have the potential to have a big impact on both how long someone lives and how well they age. We will look at a few of the ways that environmental influences may affect longevity in this post.

Air Quality: One significant environmental issue that can have a detrimental impact on longevity is air pollution. High air pollution exposure has been associated with a higher risk of respiratory illnesses, cardiovascular ailments, and other health issues. Additionally, it has been demonstrated that air pollution speeds up aging, which can reduce a person's lifespan.

Water quality: For long life and good health, access to clean water is crucial. The danger of contracting infectious diseases like cholera and typhoid fever might rise when people are exposed to contaminated water sources. Additionally, lead and arsenic exposure can have long-term health repercussions, including developmental delays and an elevated risk of cancer.

Climate Change: As a major environmental concern, climate change has the potential to have a wide range of effects on lifespan. For older persons and others with chronic health concerns, rising temperatures and extreme weather conditions, such as heat waves and storms, can be extremely dangerous. Additionally, climate change may promote the proliferation of insects that spread disease, such mosquitoes, which could increase the danger of infectious diseases.

Access to Green areas: It has been demonstrated that having access to green areas, such as parks and woods, has a good effect on longevity.

Being outside has been associated with reduced stress and better mental health, both of which can lengthen life expectancy. Additionally, green areas offer possibilities for exercise, which can lower the risk of developing chronic diseases.

Noise pollution: Exposure to loud music or traffic noise at high decibel levels can be harmful to one's health and lifespan. Chronic exposure to noise pollution has been linked to an increased risk of cardiovascular disease, cognitive decline, and sleep difficulties, all of which have an effect on general health and welfare.

In summary, environmental influences can have a substantial impact on a person's lifespan and quality of life in old age. We can contribute to the creation of better settings that promote lifespan and general wellbeing by tackling problems like air and water quality, climate change, access to open spaces, and noise pollution.

Tips For Reducing exposure to harmful toxins

There are many possible dangers in our daily life, such as pollution, toxic substances, and environmental poisons. There are steps we can do to decrease our exposure and safeguard our health, even if it is hard to totally prevent exposure to these toxins. In this article, we'll go through several suggestions for lowering our daily exposure to dangerous drugs.

Take care with the goods you use:
Numerous items we use on a daily basis, including insecticides, personal care items, and cleaning supplies, contain dangerous compounds that can be absorbed through the skin or inhaled. Consider utilizing natural alternatives, such as vinegar for cleaning or essential oils for pest management, and look for solutions that are devoid of toxic chemicals and other dangerous substances.

Increasing indoor air quality can help reduce exposure to dangerous contaminants such dust, mold, and volatile organic compounds (VOCs). Maintain good ventilation in your home, utilize air purifiers, and refrain from smoking or lighting candles or incense indoors to improve the quality of the air you breathe.

Filter your water before drinking it. Harmful elements like lead, pesticides, and medicines can pollute water. To get rid of these toxins and enhance the security and caliber of your drinking water, think about implementing a water filter system.

Consume a balanced diet: Eating a balanced diet will help you avoid being exposed to toxic substances including pesticides, heavy metals, and other poisons. Avoid processed foods that contain unhealthy additives and choose organic fruits and vegetables that are cultivated without the use of toxic pesticides.
When possible, pick less dangerous substitutes for possibly toxic products. For instance, pick low-VOC paints and finishes when painting or remodeling your home, use reusable containers rather than plastic ones, and choose natural cleaning solutions.

Use safe behaviors: Activities like smoking and drug use can expose people to toxic substances more often. Your risk of exposure to dangerous drugs can be considerably decreased by quitting smoking and abstaining from drug usage.

In conclusion, lowering exposure to dangerous drugs necessitates making decisions that are safer every day and making a conscious effort to do so. We may safeguard our health and well-being by using items carefully, enhancing indoor air quality, purifying our drinking water, maintaining a nutritious diet, selecting safer substitutes, and engaging in safe behaviors can reduce our exposure to harmful substances hence increasing our longevity.

The Benefits of Living in a healthy Environment For Longevity

The length of a person's life can be significantly increased by living in a healthy environment. A living place that promotes physical and mental wellbeing and is free of environmental toxins and risks is referred to as a healthy environment. We'll look at some of the ways that residing in a healthy environment might increase longevity in this post.

Living in a healthy environment can help decrease your exposure to dangerous things such poisonous chemicals, contaminated water, and air pollution. Exposure to these compounds has been related to a number of health issues, such as cancer, cardiovascular disease, and respiratory conditions. Living in a healthy environment can help prevent certain health issues and lengthen life by lowering exposure to these toxins.

Supporting Physical Health: There are many different ways that a healthy environment can support physical health. Better physical health can result in a longer lifetime if people have access to clean water to drink, wholesome dietary selections, and chances for physical activity. Furthermore, a healthy environment can lower risk of infection, which can affect longevity.

Promoting Mental Health: Having a healthy environment to live in can also benefit one's mental well-being, which in turn can increase longevity. The availability of green spaces, natural light, and cozy living quarters can all enhance mental health and lessen stress, which has been associated with a number of health issues. Furthermore, living in a secure atmosphere can lessen the likelihood of developing anxiety and sadness, which can impact over all wellbeing and quality.

Encouragement of Social relationships: Social relationships, which have been associated with a longer lifespan, can also be encouraged by living in a healthy environment. Access to public spaces like parks and community centers might present chances for involvement and social contact. Additionally, residing in a secure and encouraging environment can promote a sense of connection and belonging, which can improve both mental and physical health.

Supporting Long-Term Planning: Long-term planning, which is crucial for longevity, can also be supported by living in a healthy environment. Access to affordable housing, employment chances, and educational options can all help people achieve financial stability and security, which can enable them to plan for the future and lead longer, healthier lives.

In conclusion, a healthy environment can support physical and mental health, promote social relationships, and aid in long-term planning, as well as reduce exposure to dangerous chemicals. People can increase their chances of living longer, healthier lives by placing a high priority on maintaining a healthy living environment.

TECHNOLOGY

CHAPTER 8: LONGEVITY AND TECHNOLOGY

The Latest advancements in Longevity research

Recent years have seen a tremendous uptick in longevity study, with scientists and researchers from all over the world working assiduously to unearth the most recent developments in the subject. The findings of this study have the potential to fundamentally alter the way we view aging and give us the means to live longer, healthier lives. We shall examine some of the most recent developments in longevity research in this article.

Biological Genetics
The discovery that our genetic makeup influences how long we live is among the most important developments in the field of longevity study. Researchers have identified some genes, including the FOXO3 gene, that seem to be connected to a long life. Additionally, they discovered that certain lifestyle decisions, including consistent exercise, can activate these longevity genes.

Cellular Senescence
The process by which cells stop proliferating and start to accumulate damage is known as cellular senescence. Given that it can result in the disintegration of tissues and organs, this process is assumed to play a significant role in aging. Senolytic medicines, which eliminate senescent cells from the body, are one strategy being researched by researchers to prevent or reverse cellular senescence.

Restriction of Calories
A dietary strategy known as caloric restriction is lowering calorie intake while maintaining a healthy nutritional level. This treatment is now being explored in humans and has been demonstrated to lengthen lifespan in a number of animal models. The mechanisms underlying caloric restriction and its potential benefits for human longevity are being studied by researchers.
Metformin

A frequent medication for type 2 diabetes is metformin. Recent studies, however, suggest that it might also have anti-aging properties. Metformin has been shown in studies to enhance a number of aging markers, including decreasing inflammation and enhancing mitochondrial function. The potential of metformin as an anti-aging medication is now being studied.

Epigenetics
The study of changes in gene expression that are not brought on by variations in DNA sequence is known as epigenetics. The impact of epigenetic marker modifications on aging and longevity is a topic of research. For instance, they have discovered that as humans age, DNA methylation patterns alter and that these changes can be used to forecast the probability of mortality.

Secretory Phenotype of Senescence (SASP)
Cells that become senescent and start secreting pro-inflammatory chemicals experience the SASP phenomenon. It is believed that this process has a role in age-related illnesses like cancer and Alzheimer's. Senolytic medications are one strategy being investigated by researchers to block the SASP.

In conclusion, there has been substantial progress in the study of longevity recently, and researchers are hopeful that these developments will fundamentally alter how we see aging. We can create interventions that focus on these processes and potentially lengthen healthy lifespan by understanding the fundamental causes of aging. The future of longevity research appears promising, and we may anticipate seeing many more fascinating developments in the years.

How technology is changing the field of longevity

The field of longevity has been undergoing a revolution in recent years, thanks in large part to advancements in technology. Scientists and researchers are using technology to explore the underlying mechanisms of aging, develop new interventions to extend healthy lifespan, and improve the quality of life for older adults. In this article, we will explore how technology is changing the field of longevity.

Big Data and Machine Learning

Advancements in big data and machine learning have enabled researchers to analyze vast amounts of data and identify patterns that would be impossible to detect otherwise. This technology has been particularly useful in identifying the genetic and environmental factors that contribute to aging and developing interventions to target these factors.

For instance, scientists have utilized machine learning to pinpoint particular genes linked to long life and forecast how various genetic differences effect lifespan. Big data has also been used to study environmental issues like air pollution that accelerate aging and create solutions to lessen their impact.

Technology for the Body

The way we measure our health and activity levels has been changed by wearable technologies, such as smartwatches and fitness trackers. These gadgets may monitor a variety of parameters, including heart rate, sleep patterns, and number of steps walked, and they can give us information about our general health.

Additionally, wearable technology is being used by researchers to track the health of senior citizens and create interventions to enhance their quality of life. For instance, they've created wearable sensors that can recognize falls and alert caregivers, reducing the risk of injury.

Telemedicine and Telehealth

In recent years, telehealth and telemedicine have grown in popularity, especially in the wake of the COVID-19 pandemic. These technologies make it possible for medical professionals to give care remotely, enhancing older individuals' access to healthcare and lowering their risk of contracting infectious diseases.

The development of interventions to enhance the health of senior citizens has also used telehealth and telemedicine. For instance, scientists have created tele-rehabilitation systems that let senior citizens take part in physical treatment from the convenience of their own homes.

Biotechnology
Biotechnology developments have created new opportunities for creating therapies that increase healthy lifespan. For instance, scientists are looking into the potential of gene editing technology, like CRISPR, to change genes linked to aging and lengthen healthy lifespan.
The creation of novel medications and therapies to treat disorders associated with aging is another benefit of biotechnology. Senescent cells, which play a role in aging and age-related disorders like Alzheimer's and cancer, have been the subject of study that has resulted in the development of senolytic medications, for instance.

As a result, technology is fundamentally altering the study of longevity. It is enabling researchers to investigate the underlying causes of aging, create novel interventions to prolong healthy life, and enhance the quality of life for senior citizens. The future of longevity research appears bright, and even though there is still much to learn, we may anticipate seeing a lot more fascinating advancements in the years to come.

The future of Longevity and Healthy Aging

The future of longevity and good aging appears more promising than ever as technology and medical developments continue to grow. There is a growing understanding that our quality of life may be considerably enhanced as we age, with an emphasis on aging as a treatable condition rather than an unavoidable decline. We shall look at what the future might hold for longevity and healthy aging in this essay.

Individualized Medicine
The creation of tailored medicine is one of the most exciting areas of longevity research. This strategy tries to pinpoint the distinct genetic and environmental elements that cause aging and create therapies that are specifically targeted at these elements.

Researchers are able to pinpoint particular biomarkers linked to aging and age-related disorders by using cutting-edge technology like genomics and proteomics. With the help of this data, more effective and risk-free therapies and interventions can be created than with a one-size-fits-all strategy.

Medical Regeneration
Another field of research that holds out a lot of hope for the future of longevity and healthy aging is regenerative medicine. In this method, damaged tissue or organs are repaired or replaced using stem cells or other specialized cells, enabling a more thorough recovery from illness or injury.

Stem cells may be used to repair damaged tissues in the heart, brain, and other organs, according to research. This might delay aging-related decline and increase healthy lifespan.

Machine intelligence
The potential for artificial intelligence (AI) to enhance the quality of life for older individuals is enormous. AI is already making notable advances in healthcare. AI-powered systems can be used to track health status and spot disease early warning indications, enabling prompt treatment and prevention.

AI can be used to anticipate results, improve care plans, and create more individualized treatments. AI can examine enormous volumes of data and find patterns that would be impossible to find without the usage of big data and machine learning.

Behavioral Interventions

While technological and medical developments will undoubtedly play a significant part in the future of longevity and healthy aging, lifestyle changes will also be extremely essential. having a balanced diet, doing frequent exercise, and managing stress can all contribute to healthy aging and extend lifespan.

In order to increase healthy longevity, researchers are looking into the possibility of dietary and lifestyle changes including calorie restriction and intermittent fasting. These therapies have been demonstrated to lessen inflammation and enhance metabolic health, two important variables in aging and age-related disorders.

In conclusion, with potential developments in personalized medicine, regenerative medicine, artificial intelligence, and lifestyle interventions, the future of longevity and healthy aging is looking bright. In the years to come, we can anticipate even more fascinating advances as we continue to learn more about the fundamental mechanics of aging. The ultimate objective is to increase lifespan while also enhancing quality of life as we age, enabling us to experience life to the fullest.

CHAPTER 9: CONCLUSION

We now have a better knowledge of what it takes to live a long and healthy life as we come to the end of our exploration of the art and science of longevity. We can take charge of our health and lengthen our lives through a combination of scientific research and lifestyle changes.

We now know that a person's ability to live a long life is influenced by several factors, including their surroundings and way of living. With the appropriate information and resources, we may make decisions that will benefit our health and wellness.

It is crucial that we keep advancing the study of long life and good aging as we go forward. We must keep making investments in science and technology that help us comprehend the fundamental causes of aging and create efficient cures.

The art of longevity, however, can also be found in the little decisions we make every day. Healthy aging depends on our decision to put our health first, eat a balanced diet, exercise frequently, control our stress, and value our relationships.

In the end, the road toward mastering the art and science of longevity is something we must do with purpose and intention. It necessitates a dedication to self-care, growth, and learning throughout one's life. We go on this path not only for ourselves but also for the people we care about and the environment we live in.

Let's therefore embrace the art and science of aging with open hearts and minds, understanding that every step we take toward a healthier, happier life is a step toward a brighter future for both our generation and the one to follow.

21 DAYS HEALTHY HABITS JOURNAL

DAY	HABITS	REMARKS

Made in the USA
Monee, IL
02 June 2023